12.99

About the Author

Bill Longridge was born in Ireland but moved to live in Australia during the 1960s where he was to develop a deep and enduring interest in the psychospiritual. Following a successful career in business, he experienced a major life struggle in his early 40s when, as he describes it, 'Not only did I discover I'd been climbing the wrong ladder, but the ladder itself had been leaning against the wrong wall!' What was essentially an existential crisis resulted in a significant reappraisal of values, a return to his native Ireland and the decision to train in the field of psychotherapy.

Following a decade of working in private practice as an Integrative Therapist, Bill's activities today are primarily centred around his writing and the presentation of Personal Development Training for individuals, groups and organisations. In recent times, Bill has pioneered specialist personal growth training for disabled persons.

An international presenter of workshops, Bill is committed to promoting a more caring, enlightened and loving humanity. He deeply and passionately believes that the 'shedding of love's light onto darkness' provides many of the answers to the needs and problems of individuals, society and the world today.

OUT *of* PAIN *into* POWER

An inspirational guide to
life, love, happiness and success

BILL LONGRIDGE

RIDER

LONDON • SYDNEY • AUCKLAND • JOHANNESBURG

1 3 5 7 9 10 8 6 4 2

Copyright © Bill Longridge 1999

The right of Bill Longridge to be identified as the Author
of this work has been asserted by him in accordance with
the Copyright, Designs and Patents Act, 1988.

All rights reserved. No part of this publication may be
reproduced, stored in a retrieval system, or transmitted in
any form or by any means, electronic, mechanical,
photocopying, recording or otherwise, without the prior
permission of the copyright owner.

First published in 1999 by Rider,
an imprint of Ebury Press, Random House,
20 Vauxhall Bridge Road, London SW1V 2SA
www.randomhouse.co.uk

Random House Australia (Pty) Limited
20 Alfred Street, Milsons Point, Sydney,
New South Wales 2061, Australia

Random House New Zealand Limited
18 Poland Road, Glenfield,
Auckland 10, New Zealand

Random House South Africa (Pty) Limited
Endulini, 5A Jubilee Road,
Parktown 2193, South Africa

Random House UK Limited Reg. No. 954009

Papers used by Rider are natural, recyclable products made
from wood grown in sustainable forests.

Printed by The Guernsey Press Co. Ltd,
Guernsey, Channel Islands

A CIP catalogue record for this book
is available from the British Library

ISBN 0-7126-7070-X

Dedication &
Acknowledgements

To my wonderful daughters Kieran and Sharon, and their truly special mother June.

And with grateful thanks to all those significant others who have played a part in my life journey (in chronological order):

Mum, Dad, Lynda, Sam and Dougie.

The two Georges, Colin McClelland and Babs Turner.

David and Rosie Paterson, Sylvia and Tim Gaunt.

Joe and Joan Shaw, Vera and Jack Roberts.

Izzy and Alan Mattinson, Kenny and Di Bailie.

Sir Jonathan Wild, George and Cheryl Grbic.

Tony and Michelle Izzard, Marie Merrison and Tom Toomey.

Tony Cummins, John Bonney, Lenny Bourke.

Peter Nicholls and Di Nicolas.

John Turner. Len and Joan Petzer.

Maureen and Stefanie Watson. Andrea Boyd.

David and Siv Brookes. Mary Murphy, Christie and Joan McCallister.

Izzy Martin and Brian Robinson, Sr Margaret McStay, Mandy Langford and Terry Brougham.

Stef Callaghan, Bernie Shaw and Helen McClelland.

Tim Beattie. Joan Clancy. Michael and Jean Withers.

Jeff Calvert and his great keyboard skills.

Joe Heaney, Mark Reynolds, Brian Little and Harry Reid.

… And everyone with whom I've had the privilege of working as a therapist or trainer. All, in their own special way, have contributed to this book.

Special thanks go to my editor Judith Kendra and to Sonia, a truly beautiful person, for all her encouragement and support.

Dear Fellow Traveller,

Each of us breathes, lives and walks, not in the world but in our own highly individual world.

Alongside someone walking with peacefulness, we find another battling with inner conflict. Rubbing shoulders with persons strong in self-belief, we discover others imprisoned by self-doubt. There are those who feel greatly loved, whilst others perceive their lives as loveless.

The individual life path is indeed truly unique. Whilst we all are given the opportunity to 'beat our own drum and sing our own song', too often the life music we produce can cause us much distress. For many of us on this journey, our time spent upon the planet can bring great emotional pain and struggle. But as we progressively learn to travel the path of higher wisdom and love, our lives begin to heal and we step *out of pain and into power*.

Evolving towards our Higher Nature,

- our desires can translate into reality
- our isolation becomes connectedness
- our failures can be supplanted by success
- our emptiness is filled up with love
- our lives become more peaceful.

OUT *of* PAIN *into* POWER is a book of insights, inspirations and guidance – a book to help liberate our lives and set us free.

As you explore OUT *of* PAIN *into* POWER, I trust you will come more intimately face to face with the love that you truly are. And that the shedding of love's light onto darkness will help release your burdens and connect you to the source of all power ... so you can dance to the music of the Universe.

Much love and blessings,

Bill Longridge

Climbing Life's Mountains

To arrive at the summit of our potential, we all must face and conquer the many life obstacles which at times, like imposing mountains, we find standing in our way.

Any range of mountains, viewed only as a whole, can appear forbidding, even overwhelming. But, as experienced climbers know, the way to conquer a mountain range is one focused climb at a time. Gaining mastery over lower peaks, we become increasingly strengthened, building and developing confidence to face the higher and more challenging tests.

So, tackle your personal life mountains one focused ascent at a time, accurately and wisely determining over which to gain mastery first. Then, one gentle step at a time, place one foot ahead of the other. Determinedly stay on your course and soon your glorious summit will come clearly into view.

But, as you undertake each part of your journey, be sure to pause from time to time to take in and appreciate the view.

Crisis into Opportunity

To experience a transformed new self, a snake must shed its old skin. This is a highly vulnerable time for the snake, but essential to an evolved new form.

As we ourselves grow and evolve, shedding our old skins, we too may have times of crisis. At such times we can feel very vulnerable, maybe uncomfortable with life and ourselves, more than a little fragile and lacking in personal power. But we are equal to any growth crisis or it would not have been placed upon our path.

Looking closely and deeply at our crisis, we often will find hidden beneath its murky waters a jewel in the mud, a diamond disguised as adversity. As we glimpse this precious jewel, we become aware that when crisis comes along it leads opportunity by the hand.

Look for the opportunity contained within each and every crisis.

Chaos and Disorder

Chaos, confusion and disorder can sometimes be a necessary stage before we eventually arrive at higher order in our lives.

Just as when old buildings are being knocked down so they can make way for the new, so we too must sometimes endure the temporary disarray of life. Putting up with the mess and the rubble is simply a part of the process before we can enjoy our new construction.

But underneath the apparent disorder there lies an incredible intelligence, putting perfectly and solidly in place the foundations of a higher design.

Chaos, confusion and disorder are not necessarily a sign that your world is falling apart, they may mean that it is actually coming together in an amazingly wonderful way which will later be revealed.

A Wilderness Experience

We are allowed to go into the wilderness,
not so that we might lose ourselves,
but so that we might actually find ourselves,
in a more evolved and enlightened way.
And when lost and alone in life's desert,
the one who gave you water from the well,
was divinely placed upon your path.
And through that struggle of your darkest night,
you never were or ever will be
alone.

Adverse Circumstances

By closely observing life's difficult experiences, we may come in time to recognise that nothing is ever totally wasted. From the vantage point of higher meaning, at a minimum there is always learning in even the most adverse situation.

By looking for each valuable lesson we can often ease our burden of pain, as healing insights become revealed and higher understanding unfolds. Asking 'What has this come to teach me?', we are often able to transform even the most unpalatable experience into a glorious opportunity to grow.

Hidden behind the mantle of adversity we often discover the most valuable lessons, gifts masquerading as problems, to help us to heal and evolve.

Blue Skies Beyond

Just beyond the greyest of clouds
there are always clear blue skies.
Whilst the darkest part of the night
comes just before the new dawn.
And often the most colourful rainbow
will follow a tempestuous storm.

Emotional Pain

Before we can truly share the burdens of another human heart, we ourselves must first have known pain and the sorrow it can leave in its wake. Only when we ourselves have suffered does something inside us soften, enabling us to be better able to help heal others' lives.

So the emotional pain we experience is the breaking of the shell which confines our caring nature. Our exposure to emotional suffering awakens our potential for empathy and our capacity to really love. Pain reveals, expands and develops our compassionate and sensitive self.

In seeking our way out of pain, we evolve towards our higher nature, with greater understanding and a less judgemental mind. Within our pain is the gift of refinement. It seeks to mould and shape us so our true inner beauty is set free.

As pain breaks through our defensive layers, releasing the love deep within, we discover we've not been breaking down … we've actually been breaking through.

Sadness, Hurts and Loss

The expression of sadness and grief is an essential part of our wholeness. When we wall our pain inside, we are unfortunately unable to heal.

Also, wearing a mask of stoic invulnerability cuts us off from emotional support, leading to isolation and unnecessary additional pain.

The pain-producing belief that 'vulnerability equals weakness' stops others from really knowing us and inhibits the emergence and expression of the most tender parts of ourselves.

To know true emotional intimacy, it is essential to drop the veneer that we are somehow impervious to pain. Pain and sadness are integral to our humanness and by revealing where we're really hurting we let others into our heart. Big boys and girls do cry … if they wish to enjoy sound emotional health.

Tears are not only healing, they are also a living testimony to the soft and beautiful centre which lies at the core of us all.

Going beyond the Problem

If we should find ourselves becoming stuck with a difficult or stubborn life problem, we can empower ourselves to solve it by first *going beyond the problem* in the stillness of the mind.

This can readily be accomplished by holding a clear mental picture of ourselves as already having mastered our difficulty. Thus, we experience first on the inside how we want things to be on the outside.

Next, we need to act with confidence and belief, anticipating that our highest good will soon unfold in our lives. Combined with positive expectations, this creates a vibration of transcendence, strongly imprinting on our consciousness the blueprint of our future success.

So, during your darkest and bleakest night, act like the veil had already lifted, as though the dawn of new beginnings had already arrived.

Remember, when you're up against a brick wall, you're in the very best place to climb it and discover for yourself the possibilities on the other side.

Loss of Love

Life does not invite us to love in order that we might lose.

But we are sometimes destined to lose in order to gain a richer and fuller understanding of the true and deeper meaning of love.

Past Wrongs

For so many of us life is difficult and it certainly can bring with it much distress and pain.

Few of us can successfully avoid at least some times of quiet desperation, those emotionally painful periods which often are the consequence of close but bruising relationships.

But as our deepest hurts become healed, we may experience a shift in perception, a change in how we view those past painful happenings. Sometimes we may even discover that the 'wrong' inflicted upon us has proven to be a powerful catalyst that led to future healing
and growth.

Eventually we may come to recognise that our whole life has been a journey towards wholeness, a healing spiritual metamorphosis which leads eventually to unconditional love.

Forgiving Others

Forgiveness is a gift we give ourselves, as the life we heal when we forgive is our own. Forgiveness is the Royal Road which leads us to peace of mind.

By refusing to let go of past hurts, we bind ourselves emotionally to the object of our unforgiveness. Choosing to forgive another is then a choice to love ourselves.

Forgiveness begins with a decision and is a conscious act of will. However, forgetting might take some time.

Often the first essential step in forgiveness is the safe and full release of our anger. By letting out the rage we feel inside, we honour that part of ourselves which has been violated, wounded and hurt. However, the strong emotional charge of our anger can be safely and adequately released in total privacy and on our own. There is no need to damage others with our anger. When our anger has been safely discharged we are then better placed to forgive ... to release the past and let it go.

Release all resentment and unforgiveness. In so doing, you will set yourself free.

Revenge

Whilst travelling in a jungle one day, two men were suddenly bitten by a highly venomous snake. One man became so hostile that he angrily pursued the snake, determined to have his revenge. But as he doggedly chased after the snake, the poison spread throughout his body. Soon he began to grow weaker, but he refused to give up the hunt. Committed to taking his revenge, relentlessly the man kept going, but eventually he collapsed and died.

But while he had been pursuing the snake, his companion had immediately sought help. Soon he had totally recovered and was restored to the fullness of health ...

If ever you should be bitten by one of 'life's poisonous snakes', it is wise not to be consumed by the idea of revenge. The toxic venom of revenge can poison our entire being, destroying our peace of mind and filling us with bitterness and hate.

It is better to let go thoughts of revenge than to put yourself at risk.

Repeating Patterns

Our failure to learn from past errors means we
probably are destined to repeat them.

So check carefully for repeating life patterns,
recurring painful or adverse experiences. These
may be unlearned lessons from the past, again
being presented in the classroom of our lives –
further trials being placed upon our path to help
us learn and grow.

Look closely for the learning gift within painful, or
adverse, situations which keep repeating.

Difficult Times

The story is told of an unhappy Eastern prince who was going through some painful times. Things just were not going right and he was suffering a great deal of conflict and much emotional distress.

So he commissioned the royal jeweller to create a special piece of jewellery, one which would help him through these difficult days and remind him there would be better times ahead.

The royal jeweller set about the task, then some several weeks later returned to the royal palace with a simple and plain gold ring.

'I fail to understand,' said the prince, 'how this simple, albeit beautiful, gold ring can provide the reassurance that I seek.'

'Sire,' replied the royal jeweller, 'look inside the ring and there you will find inscribed three wise and important words.'

So the prince picked up the ring and there indeed were inscribed three wise and supportive words.

'IT WILL PASS' was the message for the prince ... and eventually it always does.

What to Overlook

One of the master skills of life and of all human relationships is knowing what to challenge … and what to overlook.

Exercise sound and prudent judgement.

Facing Mistakes

By refusing to face our mistakes, we are seeking to avoid our pain. But denial and self-deception can cause even greater pain.

Avoiding looking at our life errors, we fail to learn and grow and may attract similar future experiences, placed upon our pathway to help us heal and evolve.

If our error involved causing someone hurt, we may experience strong feelings of guilt. Sometimes that guilt can prove too painful to face, so that rather than resolve our conflict, we push our guilty feelings aside. If this happens, we run the risk of burying our guilt alive. And feeling 'guilty' deep in the unconscious, we might then unknowingly sabotage our happiness and highest good.

With the best of intentions and most loving of hearts, at times we all get things wrong. So, face mistakes quickly, honestly and bravely. Do all you reasonably can to heal past hurts and wrongs. Then, forgive yourself totally, and courageously move ahead towards your highest calling in life.

Carrying Past Burdens

'We must learn to release our past,
So the present is not destroyed.'

One day while walking in the wilderness, an old monk and a young monk came to a fast raging stream. Sitting there was a frightened old woman who begged them to help her across.

The vows of the monks' holy order forbade the touching of any female. However, greatly moved by the pleadings of the woman, they agreed to help her across.

So they carried her to the other side, where she thanked them and went on her way. The monks too proceeded on their journey.

Several hours later, the young monk turned to the old monk and said, 'About that old woman...'

'What old woman?' replied the old monk.
'Are you still carrying her? I put her down a long time ago...'

How needlessly we carry past burdens. To be fully alive in the present we need to let go of the past.

Learning from Mistakes

A wise man learns from his mistakes, even more than he does from his success.

But a wiser man learns even more from the mistakes that others have made.

Relativity of Problems

In a small remote village high up in the mountains, the chief elder became very distressed as so many of the villagers were coming to him with problems.

Each villager, absorbed deeply in their own struggle, considered their problem to be worse than that of any other.

Having carefully considered the situation, the elder invited his people to a meeting around a big tree located in the village square. He then requested each villager to seriously consider their problem and having done so to write it down.

'Then,' said the elder, 'all of you, pin your problem to the tree.'

He next requested each villager in turn to make their way over to the tree and read each and every one of the problems. Then, if they desired, they could exchange their particular problem for the problem of any of the others.

Having read everyone else's problem, each person decided to keep their own.

Everyone is your Teacher

See everyone you interact with in life as being purposely placed upon your path to help you, to guide you or to teach you.

By keeping constantly in your awareness that everyone is your teacher, you are then able to grow from every significant experience.

One Tree is not a Forest

Who among us with a poisoned toe would claim
our whole body is no good? Yet, when some
aspect of our experience is not quite right, how
readily we can declare our whole life to be
hopelessly wrong.

Whatever your present life struggle, constantly ask
the question: 'What's good about my life right
now?' And, if trouble should come along, be
careful not to fall for the trap of turning one tree
into a forest.

Convert your mountains into molehills.
Always look for the good and expect the very best.

Through a simple shift in perception, miracles can
often occur.

A Remedy for Self-Pity

A wonderful healing remedy for self-pity is to give some pity away.

By helping others we help ourselves.

Rigidity

Being rigid and inflexible can cause us a lot of pain. Indeed, the rigid unyielding mind can be a major source of distress.

An unbending inflexible attitude can threaten, even destroy, the most precious of relationships and many a promising business has perished on the rocks of rigidity.

A rigid unbending mind has fixed and limited vision, seeing only black and white. Sadly it fails to observe that the world is actually filled with very many shades of grey.

Life asks, 'Are you willing to sacrifice your peacefulness, to surrender your priceless life joy, upon the altar of inflexibility? Would you rather be right or be happy?'

Better to bend like the reed than be rigid like the rock. Be flexible.

Bless your Adversary

To hate, despise or curse another human being is also to wage a war within ourselves.

There is another way. We can call an amazingly potent weapon into play: love.

When we love and bless our adversary, we establish around ourselves a formidable shield of protection and also mystically set in place unseen forces of power.

Time Traps

Time can easily become a trap if we spend too much time in the past or too much time in the future.

Remaining mentally stuck in the past, we immobilise ourselves in the present, suffering regrets, guilt or self-blame – all unnecessary burdens life does not demand that we carry.

Or, filled with doubts, we look to the future and ask ourselves the question: 'What if...?' Then our anxieties come tumbling in and we begin to fill up with fear. Or we perpetually postpone actually living with the eternal promise 'Someday I'll...'

If you find yourself emotionally struggling, pause and ask yourself the question: 'Which time zone am I presently in?' Then, refuse to let the past or the future contaminate your precious present.

The past is for learning and growing, the future is for wise and prudent planning. And the present, only the present, is for being fully alive.

The pathway to the future we seek is through learning to effectively function in the precious *now* moment of time.

Non-Resistance

Water is a powerful yet non-resistant element. It does not seek to drive through obstacles, instead it flows around or over them, taking the path of least resistance.

Our strong emotional resistance to inescapable life situations only gives them greater power to cause distress. Our resistance creates an inner tension, generating fear and emotional pain.

Our lives become very much easier when we choose to stop swimming upstream, instead going with the flow of each experience.

Whilst none of us can know what we'll find around the corner, we can however let go and trust the process of life. In time, we can learn to accept that Higher Intelligence really does know best and that all will eventually unfold for our ultimate highest good.

By not judging our life situations as either good or bad, we can neutralise our resistance and relax into each experience.

The Precious Present Moment

Travelling along a wilderness way, a trekker had reached the side of a cliff when suddenly he lost his footing and went tumbling over the edge. Mercifully, while he was falling, he managed to grab hold of a vine which miraculously halted his fall.

But then, having clung on desperately for some time, he saw some rats appear and begin chewing through the vine. The man could clearly see that in a while the vine would break. Soon he would fall into the abyss.

Even in this desperate situation, he observed a wild strawberry growing out of the side of the cliff and took some precious moments to appreciate the beauty of its form. Then gently, oh so gently, he plucked the ripened wild fruit and savoured the most succulent strawberry that he ever had enjoyed …

Disengaging from the future and the past, we free ourselves to be alive in the present. Only then can we truly experience the sweetness and the riches contained in the sacred now.

The Power of Choice

One of the greatest powers in our lives is the power of choice. Through the exercise of free will and choice we have been given a freedom and dominion. We are often able to choose to walk through one of several available life doors.

Choice is a powerful facilitator through which we can be wonderfully liberated to create a new and more meaningful future. For the most part, our present life reality reflects earlier choices we have made.

However, at times we can stay needlessly restricted should we fail to recognise all our choices. Identifying all our available choices can in itself be highly liberating and can significantly reduce the tension around unsatisfactory existing conditions.

If your current life seems somewhat limited, or perhaps lacking in fulfilment, identify each and every choice that is available. Then, using wise and careful judgement, choose which door you will walk through to accomplish your highest good.

Change and Loss

'No man is an island,
If we try to live as though we are,
We can end up all at sea.'

The joyful, purposeful life path brings a necessary involvement with others, as it is only through relationships that we really get to know ourselves. Meaningful and involved living therefore brings some unavoidable dependence upon others.

But everything outside ourselves is subject to change and loss. This necessarily must include human beings who often do not change in the direction we would like. This reality can make us susceptible to relationship loss in our lives.

Being vulnerable to change and loss is an inescapable consequence of our natural interface with life.

A real acceptance of this difficult reality helps us not feel personally victimised when change or loss does occur. And it helps avoid the incremental pain which comes as a consequence of resistance to the flow of change in our lives.

The CAD Principle

We can save ourselves much pain and distress by applying the CAD principle to our lives.

It simply says:

C Change the things you can change.
A Accept those things you cannot change.
D Develop the wisdom to know the difference.

Self-Responsibility

To experience the fullness of life we must depart from the land of blaming. It is via the 'self-responsibility bridge' that we discover our promised land. Without the full acceptance of responsibility, our lives will always be limited and significantly lacking in power.

Abdicating responsibility for our lives keeps us stuck in the state of victimhood, bogged down and feeling powerless in the quicksands of resentment and blame. And when we blame others for our struggles, we make them responsible for our happiness, thus robbing ourselves of power and keeping resentment and anger alive.

Blaming looks to the past and points the finger of condemnation; responsibility looks to the future and lets us enter through freedom's door.

Ill winds can blow across our lives, but through the power of self-responsibility, we can control and master our sails.

The acceptance of self-responsibility is the passport to freedom and power.

Self-Acceptance

Self-rejection lies at the heart of much of our emotional pain. If we have to 'earn' parental love as children, we understandably come to believe that our worth resides *outside ourselves*, in what we have, what we do or achieve, instead of who we are.

How liberating the deep understanding that our inner value is fundamental to our very existence, not requiring the validation of proof.

To accept ourselves as we are, we need to let go all self-condemnation, to approve of ourselves right now instead of waiting for some future date when we might meet some self-imposed conditions.

Self-acceptance requires that we see ourselves as worthy of our own love and that we give that love to ourselves, becoming our own best friend. True acceptance calls us to recognise our own basic goodness and worth … to see the love that lies at our core.

Burning the Whip

Letting go of criticising, judging and condemning ourselves is essential to our emotional well-being. Self-acceptance, not condemnation, is the key to healing our lives.

When face to face with our mistakes, the imperfection of our humanity, it serves us all well to remember that we are here on the planet to learn.

It is important to develop 'self-nurture' – to be gentle, kind and loving towards our vulnerable and very human selves. Sadly, in most cases, no-one has hurt us more than we have hurt and damaged ourselves, through our harsh and destructive inner critic whipping our sensitive psyche.

So, wrap yourself up mentally in the warmth of your own love. Make a clear, unequivocal decision to burn and destroy for ever the cruel whip of self-condemnation.

You are a precious child of the Universe and your mistakes are merely stepping stones along your path to wholeness.

Corrective Guilt

There are times when we get things wrong, falling into error by acting without love or appropriate concern for others. At such times we may find ourselves experiencing the discomfort of corrective guilt, which rises into consciousness to instruct us, to help us be better human beings.

Corrective guilt comes along as a teacher and is not meant to be a torturer, so do not confuse its purpose. There is no need to pay endlessly for errors; all is better served by learning from our experiences.

Should corrective guilt rise into awareness, take the learning that it offers and resolve to do things better in the future. Learning from our mistakes and choosing to forgive ourselves is every bit as important as choosing to forgive others.

All of us are travelling down the same road which ultimately leads back to love.

Our Magnificent
Inner Self

'Outer beauty will fade with the seasons
Inner beauty survives for all time.'

The emergence of human personality can be likened to an emergent young rose. Contained within a young rosebud is all that is beautiful and unique. But to emerge into fullness of bloom, the rosebud needs favourable conditions like the warmth of the sun and soft falling rains. With severe and adverse conditions the flower may fail to fully open, its splendour and inner glory remaining hidden but still there deep inside.

So too with human beings. Due to adverse past conditions, or a lack of love and nurture, the bud of human personality may fail to fully open. But our true inner beauty, our wonderful authentic self, is always there deep within. Exquisite and imperishable, it needs recognition and acceptance in order to fully unfold.

Rejoice, delight and celebrate your own inner glory and magnificence, and that of all who cross your path.

Self-Respect

We need to recognise our own worth and
be willing to honour ourselves with the gift of
self-respect.

Until this has been accomplished, we remain
susceptible, even destined, to be under somebody
else's feet.

Only you can give yourself self-respect ... so do
not withhold this gift.

Our Uniqueness

The odds against someone being born exactly like you, now, in the past or in the future, are so ridiculously remote as to be unworthy of consideration. You *are* truly unique.

Many of your physical attributes are yours and yours alone. Your finger prints are unique, your toe prints are unique, your lip prints are unique, even your voice and eye patterns are distinctly and individually yours.

And, at the mental level, you are also exclusive. No-one living, dead or yet to be born will ever have exactly your thoughts. No other imagination will ever exactly compare to yours. No-one else's experience, and therefore memories, will ever perfectly match your own. And no other's life journey will ever precisely mirror the road you are destined to travel.

In so, so many ways, we are never to be repeated human beings, living an inimitable life script and on a highly individual mission.

So look with wonder into the mirror, for there you will see an image of remarkable and wondrous authenticity.

Be your Real Self

Letting go of all pretence, stepping out of our secret world and becoming our authentic self, is one of life's major milestones towards freedom.

Being our own real and authentic selves is all we ever need to be. And there really is no need to rehearse to be that truly real self, it can flow just as easily and naturally as a free-flowing mountain stream.

When we pretend to be someone we are not, the person we fool most is ourselves. Accepting ourselves, being ourselves and then 'forgetting ourselves' is the Royal Road to comfort and natural ease with others.

Hiding behind our masks only holds our pain in place as we fail to give others the chance to love and accept us as we are.

But as we discover our real self is lovable, we then become more greatly empowered to truly love and accept ourselves.

Receiving Help

Being able to give to others is, of course, very important. But equal in importance is our capacity to receive.

If we are struggling or having difficulty in life yet refuse an offer of help, we are rejecting and turning away a gift of loving service. Grateful acceptance of an offer of assistance honours both the giver and their gift of help and support.

And it is foolish to assume that others will automatically be aware of our needs. By making this assumption we can set ourselves up for pain, because if our needs are not then met, we might read this as personal rejection which can then quickly turn into resentment.

Best by far to acknowledge your needs, to recognise your own worthiness and love yourself sufficiently to ask for your needs to be met. This way, we not only value ourselves but we also value others, by providing them with an opportunity to supply a loving gift.

Open your heart to receive.

Do Not Compare

Who can make a judgement that an orchid is more beautiful than a rose; or a rose more beautiful than an orchid? There is no validity in making such comparisons; each has its own distinctive beauty.

Neither should we become deluded into comparing ourselves with others. If we do make such comparisons, we will either experience feelings of superiority or we will consider ourselves inferior and neither will serve us well.

Each one of us is here to travel a uniquely individual road. We are given our own life canvas which only we can paint. No-one else can wield our paintbrush or be allowed to mix our colours – we each must make our contribution in a way that only we can do.

So, celebrate the uniqueness of all and delight in the gift of your individual life path.

The Measurement Game

When we play the measurement game, we get to
measure ourselves against others. We get to
measure our possessions, or our achievements, or
our talents, or our intellect. We can even measure
our body if such is our desire.

But in doing so we risk 'coming up short' and this
can cause us a lot of pain: the pain of inferiority, or
inadequacy, or failure, or even of being afraid of
being 'found out'.

Participation in the measurement game can fill us
up with negative emotions: envy at what others
have, anger at what we don't have, hostility over
lost opportunities, and many many more.

So often the measurements we make are never
spoken aloud, but remain silently and painfully
inside us as destroyers of our peace of mind. For
players in this fear-based game, *wants* become
empty compensations for genuine human *needs*, as
we compare our own self-worth symbols with
those of other players.

The price of participation in this game is simply far
too high.

Feelings

In order to be wholly alive, we need to be in touch with all our feelings. The feelings which we deny are the ones which rule our lives by preventing us from being real.

And when we choose to bury our feelings, we bury them alive, not dead; they live on within the unconscious where they can produce a great deal of stress.

So, when negative feelings are triggered, don't look blamingly at another person but instead look deeply inside. Feelings arise from our perception of experiences and even the most painful feelings can bring precious healing gifts. Our painful negative emotions often point the way to our unhealed and unresolved past, our painful childhood rejections, our negative beliefs about ourselves or our areas of acute sensitivity.

But in allowing ourselves to really feel – we don't have to *act* upon feelings, by choosing to let our powerful feelings determine unwise or unloving actions.

Our feelings should not be judged as being either good or bad they are simply the carrier messengers of our deep internal experience.

Off the Hook

Letting ourselves 'off the hook' can occur when
we discover that there is no hook!

All is held in place by our beliefs. By changing the
belief, we immediately change our experience.

Making Amends

Wherever it is appropriate, it serves to consider the possibility of suitably making amends to those whom we've damaged or hurt, or from whom we've taken something away.

At times this can really be a challenge, involving us in a test of our integrity, our genuineness and our character. It can test how committed we really are to a belief in rightness and fairness, and question our sincerity and the depth of our remorse.

Making amends can also raise strong internal conflict, as our fear can sometimes step in, confronting and weakening that part of us which tells us to do the right thing. If fear should win this moral battle, our integrity becomes the loser.

But through the process of making amends, either directly if we can or indirectly through service to others, we experience the virtue of right action, simultaneously reconnecting with our inner sense of goodness. We also heal that part of ourselves which we inadvertently damaged and wounded when we unlovingly took away from another.

The Power of Listening

When you suspend your need to be heard,
enough to listen with attention and love,
you surround a person with a silence
in which they can discover themselves.
Compassionate listening heals.

Empathy

To understand the heart of another we need to walk for a mile in their shoes, to briefly experience life from their authentic point of view. Without judgement or evaluation, empathy requires that we travel, as a compassionate and loving companion, in another's highly individual world.

Empathy needs a special kind of listening where the one and only goal is the achievement of understanding, taking no account whatsoever of how we will reply. And the understanding sought is at the deeper levels of feeling, not just intellectual awareness of the other person's experience.

Empathy seeks to understand what it's really like to be this person. It listens beyond the spoken word to hear from the pain of the heart: the hurts, the losses, the regrets, the emptiness, the fears, the shame, the disappointments and the rejections.

Empathy creates a loving space in which a person can really breathe in the rarified healing atmosphere of genuine human understanding.

Empathy is a dynamic and truly powerful healer.

Non-Reaction

'Risen above offence, he could not be damaged by words.'

A truly wise guru named Sidu was famed throughout the land. People travelled from far and wide to get guidance from his words.

But a very rich merchant called Mustaq felt angry and greatly aggrieved. His two eldest sons upset him by spending time away from his business, listening to the guru's wise words.

So Mustaq decided to humiliate the wise one. Attending a gathering where he knew Sidu was teaching, he hurled great abuse at the guru.

However, Sidu remained calm and peaceful. Then he turned to Mustaq and said, 'If someone offered you a gift of poison, would you put it to your lips and swallow it?'

'Why no,' replied Mustaq.

'Neither then do I choose to swallow your poisonous offerings – I leave your gift with you.'

There is tremendous virtue and power in wisely choosing not to react to words clearly aimed to incite. Without fuel, a fire will quickly extinguish.

Quietening Anger

When someone aggressively communicates using anger, some of our best defences are:

… an empathetic listening ear
… a compassionate understanding heart
… a kind and caring smile
and
… a gentle loving response

These help form an effective shield against another person's wrath.

The Conscience

Our conscience is like the grain of sand which irritates the oyster, causing it to produce an exquisitely beautiful pearl. So, too, the human conscience agitates and irritates. It brings to our awareness our inconsiderate actions, our thoughtless selfish deeds and our uncaring and unloving ways. Through the whispers of the conscience our Higher Self speaks, inviting us to follow the rightness already known to the heart. When we ignore the voice of conscience, we ignore the teacher within, rejecting higher order for our lives.

As an instrument of evolution, which functions through correction, our conscience is ever challenging us to be our highest, most loving selves. To knowingly say 'no' to our conscience puts at risk one of life's precious gifts ... our priceless peace of mind.

However, it is essential also to recognise the important and vital difference between appropriate growthful correction and totally inappropriate feelings of guilt.

Listen with good attention to the rightness of the heart.

The Highest Choice

In our dealings with fellow journeyers, when we think and act without love, the person we wound is ourselves.

Our Higher Power knows no separation but sees us all as one, so that all we do unto others we are doing unto ourselves. So, in your daily interactions with others, make love your first and only choice. Choosing love as your guiding life principle, all that you need will be added, in perfect time and in a perfect way.

And when we choose only love for our lives, we discover a place of great safety where fears become quickly dissolved, a haven of tranquillity and peacefulness, of contentment and blissful joy.

By making love your first and only choice, you travel the highest and noblest way.

Hope

'When great hope arises within,
It attracts resources to match.'

The birth of hope is all around us. It can
be seen ...

in a tree during springtime as new buds begin to
open and fresh new leaves emerge

or in winter, when a fragile delicate flower fights to
break through the hardened earth on its journey
towards the light

or in the dawn of each new day, as golden rays
of sunlight brighten a darkened sky heralding
new beginnings.

Hope, oh glorious hope! Hope is fundamental to
the natural order and if we look through eyes
which can see, we will discover it everywhere.

Hope is one precious gift we should never take
away from another. It may be all that person has.

Apology

Move quickly to mend your broken fences. Act diligently to repair emotional hurts. Refuse to let wounds deepen due to stubborn neglect or pride. Failure to do so can cause significant loss.

A genuine heartfelt apology gives back something that was taken away. It honours a person's sense of being wronged and helps renew and restore the violated part of the self. And a genuine apology can take away so much distress, like a piercing sword removed, such is its power to heal.

An apology demonstrates both courage and character and helps restore harmony to our lives. As old wounds from the past become healed on the sacred ground of forgiveness, we all are able to return to loving and restoration of peace of mind.

So, should we regrettably or inadvertently hurt another, we can appropriately and sensitively hold forth a reconciling gift of love through the offer of our apology.

Right Actions

Always seek to do only unto others as you would have them do unto you. Know that what you give out determines what you will receive. If someone treats you harshly or unkindly, try first sending them back love instead of hate. Touched by love's invisible power, even the greatest of conflicts can be dissolved.

But it is also important to establish clear and well defined boundaries, knowing where you start and being clear about where others must end. And always send out loudly the message of your uncompromising non-negotiable self-respect.

Honesty

When we speak, or act, without honesty, we violate that part of ourselves which knows the rightness of all.

Only a life which is lived with honesty allows us to really experience a deep comfort and ease within. An honest person feels safe inside and can look comfortably into the eyes of any other, supported by the knowledge and confidence of knowing there is nothing to hide.

In the absence of honesty, we may know the unease and distress that are often companions to deceit.

We need to care and love sufficiently to be honest in all our dealings so that neither we nor others become victims of deceit.

Cherish honesty as you would a treasure of gold.

Another's Pain

In terms of finite and absolute meaning, and
totally accurate description, we can never fully
understand another's pain.

But we can lovingly support them through it.

Along your Way

Treat everyone you meet with kindness and compassion.

Remember, the seemingly least of persons is here with a gift to give.

So, whether dining in style with the rich or sharing some soup with the poor, treat all with a common dignity, courtesy and respect.

View no-one as either greater or lesser than yourself. Instead try to see all as equal; cells of one body of love.

Respect your own rights as well as the rights of others. Be tolerant of others' opinions where they differ from your own. Stay calm when confronting adversity. Keep your head in times of crisis. Take humility as your shield and courage as your sword. Fight a caring fight and run a loving race. Encourage all who cross your path.

And, throughout your Earthly mission, strive to make the planet a better place to live.

Honour your Promises

Always do the thing you said that you would do.
Keep your promises and honour your word.
And endeavour never to promise
what you know you cannot deliver.

Controlling Anger

As we witness injustice in the world, we may feel the anger of righteous indignation. Such anger can be transmuted into positive creative energy to bring about future reform.

But unbridled anger in relationships can be just like a flailing sword, chopping down all before it and at times even causing us to lose that which we have held most dear.

The greatest damage inevitably occurs when powerful charges of anger are triggered and we instantly follow our impulse to respond angrily and aggressively. But by creating a gap in time between our impulse to respond and our actual response, enflamed emotions are able to settle and a less damaging response can then be made.

However, it is better that any anger we experience be *safely and harmlessly* released rather than letting it fester and become a breeding ground for resentment and hate. The safe effective discharge of our anger can be perfectly adequately achieved in total privacy on our own, with no need to personally confront, or to violate or hurt any other.

Not Being Overly Responsible

By recognising the important difference between being responsible *for* someone and having a responsibility *towards* them, we can avoid unnecessary burdens that we really need not carry.

In adult life, we each are responsible for ourselves.

Unfair Advantage

There can be no real happiness or peace of mind through acquisition which is gained by taking unfair advantage of others or in unscrupulous ways.

Lasting happiness and durable success come from reward for honest service and can never ultimately be achieved by deliberately engaging in actions designed to create loss for others.

Make fairness and integrity the hallmark of all your dealings. Success through honest endeavour allows us to comfortably enjoy that which has been fairly acquired.

False Accusations

Malicious gossip and false accusations are two of
the most poisonous arrows we can fire at our
fellow man.

There is wisdom in establishing a rule to only say
about others in private what we would happily
have pronounced in public.

There also is much virtue in speaking only
the truth about others and that with kindness
and compassion.

And we all need to strongly resist even the subtlest
of temptations to popularise ourselves through the
sharing of dubious information.

Speak only good of others. Keep your mind
and conversation pure. This is your own best
and surest protection against the wiles of
malicious gossip.

Pleasing Others

Ostensibly, accommodating and pleasing others appears to be a healthy and loving way to function.

However, helping and pleasing others to the point of 'overhelp', or allowing ourselves to become a doormat, creates a lot of inner conflict and problems.

For pleasing others to be emotionally healthy, two primary conditions need apply. First, we need to feel comfortable and at ease with our helping, not holding inside any rising feelings of resentment. Second, helping or pleasing others should come from a place of choice and not an unhealthy place of compulsion where we feel we 'have to' please others to avoid painful feelings of guilt.

It is quite possible to unknowingly delude ourselves by thinking that meeting other people's needs is the same as meeting our own. We need to be clearly and consciously aware of the presence of our own human needs, independent of the needs of others.

If excessive pleasing others is a problem, we need to see others as being equal but not more important than ourselves.

Delight in Others

There is great blessing in the attitude that says,
'I'm so blessed that I have you in my life. Your
presence really matters and you are missed when
you're not here.' How the human heart rejoices in
the knowledge that our very existence is a source
of joy and delight to someone else.

So, when someone really matters in your world,
commit to telling them clearly how you feel.
Enrich them freely, openly and generously,
ensuring that they know for certain that their life
and presence really do make a difference.

Taking Offence

As caring human beings, we would not
deliberately set out to give offence to others.
However, where no offence has been intended, it
is just as damaging and cruel to take offence as it
ever can be to give offence.

It is important to remain alert, lest we
unknowingly use taking offence as a weapon to
hurt and punish others.

Unhealed Partners

A successful and happy relationship does not need two perfect people who are wholly emotionally healed. However, it ideally does require two people who are open and committed to their own and their partner's growth. To create a loving relationship, we need a willingness to accept and help heal the most wounded parts of ourselves and the most wounded parts of our partner.

Relationships are best served by a non-judgemental environment where emotional honesty and openness are encouraged and highly prized. And there needs to be a resolve – even sacred commitment – that the partners should not knowingly or deliberately set out to hurt or damage each other.

Be gentle, kind and loving towards your partner and yourself. Be compassionate, accepting and nurturing towards those vulnerable, fragile parts you may discover within yourself or within your significant other.

Foolish Words

When a person is speaking with wisdom,
their words will be comfortable to our ear.
But when their words are spoken in foolishness,
we will find our listening hard.

Surrendering 'Attack' Thoughts

At times we can fail to recognise our more subtle experiences of fear, which can unconsciously distort into anger, causing 'attack' thoughts against our fellow man.

But when we think and act with fear, we are emotionally attacking ourselves, wrongly mis-creating through improper use of thought.

However, we always have the opportunity to explore our feelings of anger and, looking closely to find out what lies beneath them, we can often unmask our fear. Often it is fear of inadequacy, or inferiority, or rejection, or humiliation, all being held in place by an inner lack of self-worth. So, when we surrender attack thoughts completely, we find that others haven't made us feel angry. Our anger has arisen from within by choosing fear instead of love.

We can make a clear and conscious decision to surrender all attack thoughts against others, and instead choose peace of mind, by thinking and acting only with love.

Appreciation

The expression of genuine appreciation effectively honours others and the gifts they bring into our lives.

An inability to show appreciation, on the other hand, often reflects a broader struggle with the capacity to emotionally give. When we fail to show appropriate gratitude, we unfortunately withhold from others a very important gift.

Sincere and heartfelt appreciation is a way of giving to others the affirming recognition that is the gift of a grateful heart. We all need to be acknowledged and appreciated to know that our efforts are valued and that our gifts have been worthwhile.

Each of us can reap much benefit by looking closely at our lives to make ourselves more aware of the gifts that we have received. Then openly, freely and generously, we can express the earnest gratitude of a thankful acknowledging heart.

How easy it can be not to value a gift we've been given. All too late this may come to our awareness when, alas, it's been taken away.

The Very Best Light

Three artists were requested to paint a portrait of the king, each being commissioned to create a separate work. But a problem confronted the artists: how to paint the king's imperfections, he had a hunch in his back and one partially withered eye.

The first artist showed the king as truly handsome, with an altogether perfect physique. But this exaggerated falseness angered the king and the artist was thrown into jail.

Learning of the first artist's fate, the second showed the king as really ugly, even emphasising his imperfections. Such honesty without kindness also enraged the king and this artist too was put in jail.

But the third artist won the king's favour. He painted the king shooting grouse, one eye appropriately closed, looking down the barrel of his gun, and with a natural arch in his back as he leaned across a fence taking aim …

Each of us can help our fellow journeyers by helping them see themselves in the very best possible light.

Judging Others

When even the laws of our society declare us innocent until proven guilty, what right do we have to impose our hasty judgements on each other? And who amongst us is so without error that we would be willing to cast the first stone? If we set ourselves up as judge, do we not also set ourselves up to be judged?

We all are vulnerable, imperfect, often frightened human beings, frequently the product of a damaging and painful childhood. But beyond any individual's 'dark side' is a spectre of pure light; a core of imperishable beauty. This light is the 'love essence' of man – the divine spirit dwelling within – and it can never be extinguished.

So, before condemning others for their errors, pause for a moment of reflection. Does not our attitude of condemnation itself confirm, at least to some extent, that the same potential for error might also exist within ourselves?

We can always judge another person's action without judging and condemning the person.

Loving Correction
of Others

If we can clearly see a loved one at risk of falling into a hole, is it not both responsible and loving to help them avoid that hole?

Without judgement or condemnation, is it not better to correct another in an unconditionally loving way than to have the person believe that you really do not care?

Lovingly correcting another, with tenderness and sensitivity, is certainly much more caring than flattering their error or folly.

An honest answer, delivered with kindness, is a sign of genuine friendship and much more helpful and loving than simply saying what the other wants to hear.

Hold Lightly

If our attachments in relationships become too
strong, we may find that we experience fear of loss.
This can lead us to hold on much too tightly
even risking crushing our most valued and
treasured gifts.

Holding on too tightly can place negative fearful
energy around the object of our attachment and so
put our whole relationship at risk.

Always be prepared to let go. If something
truly belongs to you, it will return. If it doesn't, it
was not meant to be permanently yours in the
first place.

Hold lightly, not tightly.

Right Ingredients

Compassion, caring and goodness are ever-present ingredients in a peaceful, joyous person.

But unkindness, cruelty and malice are never to be found where enduring happiness resides.

Masks

Don't be fooled by the masks which people wear.
The mask might look like arrogance, or aloofness,
or rudeness, or uncaringness – but behind that
mask is a person who deep down inside is afraid.
The mask is simply a defence, a wall erected by a
struggling human being seeking to avoid
future pain.

Should the mask begin to slip, behind it you will
find the uncertainty, the deeply disguised doubts,
the loneliness and the fears. The person behind the
mask needs desperately to believe they are
something, that they have value, that they are
lovable and acceptable as a member of the
human race.

No matter how ugly it may appear, the mask does
not conceal a bad person, just someone who is in
great pain. Difficult as it may be, it is your loving
unconditional acceptance which will throw
that person a lifeline, enabling them to
accept themselves.

However, before we can unmask another, we must
first learn to unmask ourselves.

Share your Learning

Generously share with others your wisdom and valuable life lessons. Be liberal with your healing knowledge where you know it could help another's life.

And if you set out to teach another, try to do so in a way that liberates. Remember, if you give someone a fish, you feed them for a day, but teach them how to fish and you will have fed them for life.

As you lovingly share your understanding, it becomes more strongly imprinted on your consciousness as whatever knowledge or wisdom you are expressing in turn becomes more deeply impressed.

Sharing precious learning with another can help comfort, support or empower one weakened and dispirited by struggle.

So, without seeking to impose your view, generously and lovingly share the healing insights you've been given.

Gentle Change

In relationships with others and life,

if something is not broken, do not try to fix it.

If a dog is sleeping peacefully, let it lie.

But if there is something that needs to be changed, do not be heavy handed but use the feather touch and be gentle as a lamb.

Responding to Another's Error

When someone is in error, respond with sensitivity and gentleness. Always be prepared to let others save face. Make sure that you leave them with their dignity still intact.

Separate the person from the problem, continuing to value the person while working on the problem. Set out to make the other's faults seem easy to correct, while making certain that self-esteem is well protected at all times,.

Endeavour to point out how things can be better in the future and refuse to dwell on a past which you know cannot be changed.

Should you need to help rectify error, seek to do so with tender compassion ideally empowering the person to face the world with strengthened self-belief.

Shaping Behaviour

In seeking to shape behaviour, you will find it helpful to remember that behaviour which is rewarded is more likely to be repeated, while behaviour which is ignored is more likely to become extinct.

It's also worth keeping in mind that receiving attention from others also constitutes a form of reward.

Avoiding Damaging Arguments

To avoid damaging and destructive arguments, agree with your adversary quickly or withdraw.

Just like a breach in a dam, an argument permitted to develop can become like a raging torrent, threatening to overwhelm all.

When powerful emotions become aroused, it is better to temporarily withdraw and allow them to settle down. Then the issue of disagreement can later be addressed in a more constructive and less damaging way.

Self-Revelation

We all have our painful inside story, shattered dreams, powerful regrets, painful rejections, shameful failures and hidden fears. But hidden secrets about ourselves, held inside, can be the source of much emotional pain.

The safe sharing of previously guarded secrets can be like the lancing of a boil, providing huge emotional relief and a lowering of internal tension. But to reveal our hidden self we need to feel really safe, as we are putting the gift of our deepest trust into the hands of another.

The sharing of our real selves with another, telling them who we really are requires us to lay bare the most vulnerable parts of ourselves. And our sharing needs be received with gentle loving tenderness, with compassion and sensitivity, and the deepest of respect.

However, having shared our pain and known the love of true acceptance by being accepted as we are, warts and all, we become wonderfully liberated and empowered to love and accept ourselves.

Acceptance of Others

By accepting someone as they are in a truly unconditional way, you 'love into' that person the power to change, to heal and transform their life, often in miraculous fashion.

Marriage

In a marriage, love each other with patience and gentleness. Try not to take your love for granted but value it like a treasured gift. Understand and pay caring attention to the needs you each will have.

Be appreciative and show gratitude freely. Allow one another to grow, supporting each other well as you both face your fears and the challenges of life.

Endeavour to maintain good humour. Always enter your home with a smile. Never be too old to hold hands and hold each other's heart with tenderness when there is the need to release inner pain.

Be careful to avoid destructive criticism, that great destroyer of human relationships. Don't let the sun go down upon your wrath but instead choose to freely forgive, avoid dragging up the past to use as a weapon in the now.

Be honest in all communications, always tempering your honesty with sensitivity, compassion and kindness. Greatly cherish the gift of trust, once broken it is hard to repair.

And say 'I love you' often.

Valuing Others

To go beyond conditional love, we must give a
greater gift than praise, valuing others for who
they are, not just for what they do.

Children

Children are the wondrous expression of life's eternal longing for itself.

Every child born is of inestimable worth. The value and worth of each child is intrinsic to its very existence and not found outside the child in what it might become or achieve. So, do not limit your approval of a child to achievements, or place harsh and severe conditions upon the lovability of your children.

Provide children with wise guidance, whilst not seeking to impose your desires upon their own unique life journey. Their life is theirs to live.

Treat every child as precious, be gentle and show much tenderness. Be a wonderful encourager, generous with your praise, patient with mistakes and a source of great inspiration.

Above all, love your children without conditions – fresh from their bath or covered with dirt, in their moments of achievement and glory or their times of painful defeat.

Tell your children often that you love them … and love them totally, always and unconditionally.

A *Smile*

A kind and loving smile is like a welcome oasis to
one parched and thirsting for kindness in a
sometimes cold and inhospitable world.

And each time we smile lovingly at another, our
heart smiles back at us and our whole being is
filled up with light.

Your kind and loving smile is a ray of warm heart
sunshine and no-one needs your smile more than
those who have none to give.

So, smile often, lovingly and generously, flooding
everyone in your world with the sunshine of
your heart.

Our Words

Be slow to speak,
quick to listen.

Place greater value on the quality
than the quantity of your words.

Our words spoken with cruelty
can be deadly as a sword.

But a word spoken in kindness
can heal a wounded heart.

Choose your words wisely.

Jealousy

Jealousy is a manifestation of deep-seated feelings of inadequacy and an exaggerated fear of loss. The tortuous experience of jealousy can cause even those held most precious to suddenly become our enemy.

But jealousy is not about another person, it is all about ourselves, and the answer to this difficulty lies within.

To heal this painful emotion, we need first to acknowledge and own our previously hidden fears. Once jealousy is 'out of the closet' and our fear is brought into the light, it can soon begin to weaken, as the ultimate strength of any fear lies within its covert nature.

If jealousy is a problem, as indeed it is for many people, do not get angry with yourself, but learn to love and accept yourself more. Learn to recognise, appreciate and value your intrinsic goodness and worth. Know that you are a special and beautiful person.

We never ever can lose that which is ours by divine design. Nothing and no-one can ever separate us from the higher plan for our lives.

The Inner Candle

No lasting happiness can ever be found by blowing out someone else's candle so that our own will burn more brightly in the world.

To do so creates within us a darkness in which we will find it more difficult to see ourselves in a loving light.

Every unkind and malicious action strips away our joy so only do unto others as you would have them do to you.

Enriching Others

The human heart longs for acceptance, for tender love and appreciation. And love is perfectly fashioned so that when we are kind and loving to others we are also being best to ourselves.

In fact, we can best provide affirming love to others by first becoming fully aware of the beauty that resides within ourselves. The more we see that beauty within ourselves, the easier it becomes to discover the beauty in others.

We also need the vision and the willingness to really look for the good in others, because at times it can be strongly masked.

Then, we need to hold still the mirror, lovingly reflecting back to others their own goodness, riches and splendour ... and their inestimable value and worth.

As we discover the beauty in others, the quality of beauty itself becomes more deeply absorbed into our own hearts and minds.

Peace of Mind

In the absence of peace of mind there can be no enduring happiness or success. So embrace your peace of mind like a precious and priceless gift, as its worth is way beyond measure.

Wherever it is possible in life, do not compromise your peace of mind, but diligently and watchfully protect it.

When facing your major life decisions, make peace of mind your perfect guide. Where you can, avoid decisions or pathways that would be destructive to a peaceful life.

Endeavour to make your peace of mind a prized and treasured jewel in your life.

Worry

No-one is born a worrier. Worry has to be learned. Often it is modelled during childhood from one or both of our parents. However, worry can also be unlearned.

Today is the tomorrow we worried about yesterday. Yesterday itself is a fast-fading shadow and tomorrow only exists in the mists of imagination. So, take no anxious thought for tomorrow, avoid the crystal ball predictions of negative imagination. Mentally, fasten each day within a tightly sealed compartment so it then does not contaminate or darken your new dawn.

Keep all your thoughts and energy focused on the things you can influence, those aspects of your life which are within your power to change, not those matters outside your control.

Take your life just as it comes – one wonderful day at a time. Let go and let the Universe take care of all the details.

Non-Resistance

Before setting off on a journey, a mountain dweller tethered his goat, fastening it securely to a tree with a lengthy piece of rope.

Soon after the man had departed, the goat began to feel fearful. It started anxiously pacing around and became hopelessly caught up in the rope. The more it struggled to get itself free, the more entangled it became. Finally, totally exhausted, it lay down upon the ground and fell asleep.

In a clear and vivid dream, the goat saw itself freed from bondage, exactly as it wanted to be. And its natural movements while asleep gradually untangled the rope, so that when it eventually awakened, it discovered that it really was free ...

So, too, through fearful thinking, we can become hopelessly entangled and disempowered. But we can release our anxiety and resistance by learning to trust and let go. Then, by holding a clear vision of life beyond our present struggles, we can put in place unseen forces and begin to set ourselves free.

Trivial Disturbances

At the beginning of each new day it pays to be still for a while to reflect upon your major life goals and your mission here upon Earth.

By making this a regular practice, any trivial disturbances which later come along will begin to lose their power to upset you. By staying oriented to the bigger picture, you will find life's annoyances and irritations, whether people or situations, quickly become inconsequential.

So, if you find yourself becoming disturbed by the minutiae of life, gently direct your focus back to your higher purpose. Soon your peace and equilibrium will be restored.

Impatience

Impatience can be the product of an anxious, restless mind. By demanding that things happen quickly, it can cause us to give up too soon. And to achieve real mastery in life, we need to make patience our friend.

Impatience can also cause loss of quality through rushing to complete a task.

And when we are impatient with others we may be lacking understanding and tolerance, by demanding they achieve completion in a time frame they might struggle to meet.

But impatience can be a response which we have learned and it therefore can also be unlearned. By frequently stepping into the role of a very patient person, acting as if you already are the most patient person in the world, you soon will be able to observe your patience beginning to expand.

You can act your way into patience by daily assuming the role of the patient person you would like to be.

Growth

We are just like a tree – as we live, we grow. Our growth is evidence of life. So, do not postpone your living, like the person of whom it was said 'buried aged 70 but died aged 30'.

Seek to live your life to the full. Treat each and every day like the precious gift that it is, grabbing with both hands every wonderful opportunity to taste exciting and growthful new experiences.

Really step into life, engaging with it fully. Embrace the myriad possibilities which can lead to joy and fulfilment.

Make your life an exciting adventure, painting your own unique canvas exactly how you want it to be.

Seek to live your life to the full.

Its Own Reward

When we understand the deeper meaning of love, we do not seek to love 'selectively', nor do we look for a return for the love that we have given. A truly enlightened person knows that the act of loving itself brings with it its own reward.

However, as we give our love freely away, it actually becomes impossible to avoid the avalanche of blessings you can be certain will return. And the more love we generously give, the more complete our lives become, as the love within us expands and our joy and happiness grow.

Our return is guaranteed. It is simply just not possible to give more than we receive, as all that we give to others, we are giving to ourselves.

Life Balance

When our life is out of balance,
just like a wheel that is not round,
it will surely travel roughly
over the ground of human experience.

Ensuring our life is structured
to incorporate healthy balance,
is one of the master secrets of bliss
supporting emotional and physical well-being.

To avoid much tension and stress,
endeavour to live your life at a pace
which is comfortable and right for you.

Strive to live a life which is balanced.

Confidence versus Faith

Confidence has its foundation in what has gone before in our lives. It looks to the past and is based upon the known.

But *faith* is trust in the unknown, in what has yet to come. Faith is our belief and trust in things we have not seen.

The whole Universe is held in place by forces we cannot see. Faith is trusting that same intelligence which holds all in perfect place.

Possessions

It simply would not make sense to put up curtains in a railway carriage whilst making a brief journey by train. Equally it makes little sense to become overly attached to possessions as we briefly walk the Earth. Not one iota of what we possess will depart this planet with us and coffins do not have pockets.

It's also useful to remember that we do not always have to own in order to enjoy. Many of life's wonderful offerings are both free and readily accessible. Like the beauty of the forest where we walk ... the restful pleasure of the beach and the sea ... the sanctified peaceful atmosphere of a serene majestic mountain.

It is so easy to become obsessed by possessions, but an unhealthy attachment to having can distort what we are becoming.

Celebrate, give thanks and enjoy all the gifts you've been given but avoid being possessed by possessions.

Fear

Fear begins as a negative thought, accompanied by negative imagination, which we erroneously judge as reality. We then anticipate that something bad, something painful, maybe humiliating, will happen to us in the future.

But there is an old Chinese proverb which says 'Fear knocked upon my door but when I opened it there was no-one there.'

Though the feelings of fear are very real, the actual fear itself is an illusion. Fear has often been rightly described as False Evidence Appearing Real.

Fear gets its strength from its darkness, from lurking in the shadows of the mind, but if you hold it up to the light it will immediately begin to weaken. By putting the false evidence of fear into the witness box for examination, we discover it cannot defend itself, as it is nothing but a trickster.

Release from fear can come by surrounding every situation with love. Perfect love will cast out fear.

Take Life Lightly

The greater our ability not to take ourselves too seriously, the lighter the burdens we will carry.

Being able to laugh easily at ourselves diminishes the probability of pain and of becoming overwhelmed by the seriousness of life. Taking both ourselves and life more lightly, we make it easier to handle adversity if and when it should happen to come along.

So, try to relax and lighten up and decide to really enjoy your time here on planet Earth. Laugh often. Celebrate and really delight in this precious gift of life, sadly, all too quickly it is gone.

Always

Always have the courage to say
when you don't know.

Always have the humility to admit
when you are wrong.

Always have the wisdom to know
when to ask for help.

Indolence and Indifference

Indolence is a much maligned, often misunderstood human condition. Often, a seemingly lazy person is caught up in emotional conflict, trapped in a web of inadequacy and plagued by fears and self-doubt. Frequently, an attitude of complacence or indifference simply masks deep-seated anxiety.

Concealing their inner feelings of worthlessness, such a person often secretly aches for a life which has meaning and purpose. The outside appearance of indifference obscures the inside experience of uncertainty, born of low self-esteem.

Typically, harsh criticism and condemnation do not serve a demotivated person who may be struggling to get just an inkling that they might have some value and worth.

The deeper healing lies in helping this person to reach a place of greater self-belief to discover that they are valuable and lovable, that they can 'make it' despite doubts and fears.

'Concentrate Easy'

In the world of physical labour, the more strenuous the effort we expend, the better the result. The harder we dig, the bigger the hole.

But in the mental world of concentration, too much stressful effort readily defeats itself. The secret of effective concentration is calm and relaxed ease, not stressing and straining to get results.

The more relaxed and at ease we are, the better our attention and focus, and the easier it then becomes to absorb and retain information or to find creative expression.

Concentrate easy, not hard.

Creation

To observe is to create

To listen is to create

To think is to create

To feel is to create

To imagine is to create

To take action is to create

To remember is to create

To forget is to create

To love is to create

To forgive is to create

To breathe is to create ...

We are in a constant state of creation.

Wise Decisions

We tend to make better decisions when we consider in advance the probable outcomes our decisions will create.

By taking a little time, we can contemplate and examine the implications of our significant decisions, and the effects our actions will have – upon ourselves, upon others or the world.

Consider carefully all probable outcomes so the wisest decision is made.

Easy Change

Every summer, a kindly gentleman farmer would invite local village families to a picnic on his land. It was held by a beautiful pond, fed by crystal-clear waters from a pure mountain stream.

But one day the water became polluted, as the pond became choked and overgrown with weeds.

The farmer examined the pond and decided that to clear it would be difficult, so he kept putting off the task. Then, finally one day, he decided to do the work. To his amazement and delight, as he began to pull out the weeds, they came away with consummate ease. He then began to really wonder why he had ever delayed the task.

To put any change in place requires the decision to make it happen. But inertia can set in if we believe that the change will be hard. By firmly installing the belief that *change is easy*, any transition in life becomes less difficult to put in place.

Correction of Knowledge

A seeker of knowledge and truth will want to
know when they are wrong.

When rightly and appropriately corrected, the
truth seeker pays good attention, not taking
unnecessary offence or erroneously interpreting
the correction as evidence of personal rejection.

A person committed to growth will always be open
and grateful for each and every opportunity which
helps them learn and grow.

Duty versus Love

If we take on responsibility for the voluntary care of another purely out of a sense of duty or to avoid inner feelings of guilt, we risk generating hostile feelings within ourselves.

Also, in such situations there exists a substantial difference between a genuine loving acceptance and an attitude of resignation. With the latter comes the prospect of resentment.

Ideally, all our caring duties should be carried out with love. However, if this just is not possible, we should not condemn ourselves or feel guilty, but simply endeavour to get help from another who can more comfortably perform the task.

Your Body

Your body is a temple in which eternal spirit dwells. It is a truly wondrous vehicle in which you travel your Earth journey, expressing the life you are here to live.

It is wisdom to honour your body and to treat it with great respect. This way it will serve you best.

So refuse knowingly or willingly to cause your body abuse or inflict upon it substances you know will cause it harm. Live a healthy lifestyle, one that would support you if you were living on a desert island with no physician close to hand.

Though we cannot know how long we will live, make your plans and set your goals for a long and healthy life. Then endeavour to look after your body in a way that will support those plans.

Love your body.

Relaxing into Trust

While flying across a desert, a young seagull became very thirsty. Endlessly it searched for water and finally was able to find some in the bottom of an old tin can wedged firmly in the sand.

Perched upon the rim, the young bird stretched and strained, but the level of the water remained just beyond its reach. Weakened and exhausted from the struggle, it finally lay down on the sand and soon was fast asleep.

In a dream, the great white gull appeared, saying, 'Have no fear. Let go and trust. I will show you your perfect way.'

When the bird eventually awakened, inspiration flooded its mind. Excitedly, it flew around the desert eagerly gathering up pebbles, then, one by one, it dropped the pebbles into the can. Soon the level of the water rose and the bird could drink its fill ...

So we too can discover our perfect way when we let go of our concerns, relax, become still and listen ... so our Higher Self can speak.

Good Grace

If assigned an unavoidable task which you feel you'd rather not do, make a clear and definite decision to do it with good grace.

Performed with bad grace and resentment, any task will become more unpleasant and often more difficult to perform.

So, do all you must do with good grace. This way you will serve yourself best.

Giving

'Generous giving creates much joy. Do not deny
yourself this gift.'

Those who haven't yet learned to really give have
unknowingly deprived themselves of one of life's
most precious gifts. Indeed, there can be no
fullness of joy without a loving willingness to give.
Our rich and abundant Universe calls us to be free
and generous givers, urging us to greater
compassion and expression of a more loving self.
And by freely giving to others, we help that loving
self to emerge.

In truth, all we give to others we are giving to
ourselves and all that we do to others we are doing
to ourselves. It therefore becomes impossible to
give without receiving. And, as we lovingly give to
others, the love within ourselves expands, filling us
up with joy.

Give and you shall receive. This is the promise of a
bountiful Universe which loves a generous giver.

Envy

Observing what others have can put us painfully and uncomfortably in touch with what we do *not* have. This unwelcome awareness can then trigger powerful unwanted feelings like inadequacy, inferiority, feelings of failure or strong regrets. So, unconsciously we then defend against this pain, by projecting our disapproval onto those who appear to have more.

Ironically, by condemning others for having we avoid condemning ourselves for not having. Thus envy, very cleverly and subtly, is a way of denying our pain.

The release of envy begins with the awareness that it is there, owning it without condemnation or harsh judgement against ourselves. By accepting ourselves as we are we make it easier for ourselves to change.

Then, by supplanting the ill-will of envy with goodwill, blessings, even admiration, we gradually become free to access our own channels of supply.

Greed

Greed is born of a fear of lack and a belief in limited supply.

It can be likened to a person terrified of being thirsty, though the well is always full and the reservoirs overflow. But such an unquenchable thirst can only be removed by recognising and owning the fear, then facing it head on.

Overcoming greed and fear of lack comes through learning to give. Gently learning to lovingly give, in time we desensitize our fear, eventually we can come to feel safe and quite comfortable with our giving.

As the mind really tastes the difference between the acrid emptiness of greed and the sweet tasting pleasure of giving it soon requires no further convincing.

A generous heart creates much joy.

Life's Coincidences

Often our Higher Power intervenes directly in our
lives through what might appear to be
coincidences, those curiously extraordinary events
which amazingly come together in a perfect way
and in perfect time.

By examining our significant coincidences, we
often are able to discover a clearly discernible
pattern, shaping and fashioning our lives in the
direction of our highest good.

Finding Truth

The ancient gods met one day to decide where they would hide Truth, as they wanted to put it in a place which would prove difficult for man to find.

One god proposed it be hidden on top of the highest mountain, while another god suggested the depths of a deep blue sea. Yet another proposed hiding Truth far in the deepest valley or maybe the unfathomable reaches of a dark and secret cave. Alas, the gods could not agree and much debate took place.

Finally, one god suggested, 'Let's hide Truth inside man – he will never think to look there.'

And all the gods agreed …

All truth lies within. Seek and you will find it, and the truth will set you free.

Over-Identification

During our Earth journey, we each play many roles in the rich and colourful theatre of human experience.

But if we become 'over-identified' with our role, we run the risk that it can take us over, causing a loss of balance in our lives. If this occurs, we may find ourselves perplexed and disturbed by the seemingly critical importance and seriousness of it all.

Retaining a healthy and balanced perspective is essential to both our emotional and our spiritual well-being. So, do not become obsessed with your role to the extent that you lose touch with your humanity or put at risk your sensitivity to the rights and needs of others.

We each are creator and director of our own unique life drama, so be sure to choose a role which reflects your higher nature and serves your highest good.

The Anonymous Gift

In terms of absolute meaning, it certainly could be argued that totally altruistic giving simply cannot exist, as any form of giving brings pleasure to the giver.

However, it is foolish to challenge our motivation to give on the grounds that giving produces pleasure. In fact, love has been perfectly fashioned so that through the act of giving itself both the receiver and the giver obtain a gift.

Our reward of warm, wonderful feelings, resulting from the process of giving, strongly supports and encourages us to become even more loving givers.

But in terms of truly selfless giving, probably the closest that we can achieve comes through totally anonymous giving.

Boredom or Adventure

Life can be dull, boring and dreary, an unexciting routine, or it can be a continuous and stimulating challenge, an ever-expanding adventure. The possibilities are truly endless ... and the choice is ultimately ours.

However, the real question for us all is which kind of life will we choose?

Choose Right Memories

There may be times in our lives, especially during healing seasons, when it is both necessary and appropriate to pay attention to our painful past.

However, in normal everyday living, we can make ourselves very unhappy by choosing to dwell upon painful memories. As we all get to choose just which memories we hold in our awareness, every one of us has the power to consciously direct our focus. Choose foolishly and we've chosen pain, choose wisely and we can bathe in empowerment.

So, if you must spend some time in the past, choose a time which serves you well, utilising resourceful memories to empower yourself in the *now*.

Live with Joy

Let your joy and laughter fill the air. We all need joy and pleasure to balance the seriousness of life.

By allowing ourselves to freely enjoy, we release the 'free child' within, letting it find rightful and needed expression. Refuse to become downcast or heavy laden. Instead, empty your heart of struggle by casting every one of your burdens onto your Higher Power. Understand, with total conviction, that nothing is impossible to those who walk with love.

Dance with a joyful spirit. Laugh often and laugh freely. Keep your countenance towards the sunshine so your life can't be darkened by shadows. Be a transmitter of cheer and goodwill. Look forward to the miracles of each day. Know that those who bring their joy into the lives of others will simply find it impossible to keep it from themselves.

And always remember well that the most beautiful things in the world cannot be seen or touched ... they need to be felt by the heart.

Prayer and Meditation

When we pray, we do the talking and call our Higher Power.

It's in the silence of meditation that our Higher Power gets to call us back.

Building
Inner Resources

Each time we confront and overcome a life difficulty, a major setback or significant challenge, our mental and emotional immune systems become more greatly empowered.

It's as if we receive an 'emotional vaccine' which strengthens and protects us mentally when a similar or bigger challenge comes along.

When we face and resolve a life difficulty we become internally more richly resourced, taking greater resilience into the future.

Through solving our life's problems, we expand our personal power.

Humility

There is wonderful virtue in humility and a person who walks with humility has evolved beyond personal vanity.

The higher lessons of humility teach that we are the precious instrument but not the instrument maker. When such a recognition combines with surrender of our lives to Higher Will, we then can be used as an instrument of great power. The more we embrace humility, the greater work we will be called upon to do.

Humility creates a protective shield. Others do not attack a humble person as they might a person all puffed up by pride. Humility also brings an increased confidence. Not having placed itself up high, there is much less fear of a fall.

There certainly exists no conflict between a life that is lived with humility and a healthy valuing of the self.

Humility brings with it great attractiveness – how readily a humble person can comfortably find a place in our heart.

Seek
Self-Understanding

Seeking to really understand ourselves is certainly
not mandatory in life. However, it is an essential
precursor to freedom ... and an unexamined life
will rob us of great riches.

Our Beliefs

We look out at the world through the window of our beliefs. If that window is stained and streaky it will distort our view of the world.

But we don't look out at the world and see things *as they are*, we see things *as we are*. Our world is a mirror of our beliefs, accurately reflecting back what is going on inside ourselves. The self-limiting beliefs which we hold create negative and fearful expectations and cause us to make negative interpretations of events going on in our lives. And what we ultimately do with our lives will be determined by the beliefs which we hold.

However, we can release old beliefs from the past which have imprisoned us and caused us pain. Positive change can quickly occur by letting go of all disempowering beliefs: about ourselves, others or the world.

And a belief is only a thought, an idea held on to with conviction. Change that thought and you can dramatically change your life ... and discover that you are not limited.

Be Magnanimous

Be magnanimous; give generously back to life.

The more we return to life of the gifts that we've been given, the more additional gifts we will receive.

So, willingly give two loaves to the beggar who asks for one: he is actually your paymaster in disguise.

Never miss an opportunity to give or to be of loving service. Such opportunities simply make it possible to give a loving gift to yourself.

All that we give to others, we are giving to ourselves.

Our Point of Power

It is easy to fall into the trap of postponing important change in our lives.

But our point of power is ever with us, vested in each new moment. So, any new moment in time can become *our* moment of decision, setting in place unseen forces and the energy of transformational change.

However, the real question which challenges us all is: How long will we delay that moment?

Do not delay your highest good.

The Courage to
Rise Higher

Take great courage and expand your horizons. Go
to the edge of your previous limitations ... and rise
higher than you've ever gone before.

Through courage, boldness and confidence, we
can overcome the fear which keeps us bound and
imprisoned, circumscribed by limitations.

When we look for the hero inside ourselves, we
invariably will discover powerful inner resources
we did not even know were there.

Step out boldly and in faith never wavering: your
Higher Power will empower you to successfully
carry out the work appointed for you to do.

The Power of Dissatisfaction

One of the primary preconditions for change is the presence of dissatisfaction when we know, deep down inside, that something in our lives is not quite right.

Dissatisfaction creates inner conflict which calls out for resolution, like a strong internal tension which needs to be relieved. Whilst dissatisfaction is often viewed negatively, it can and does provide powerful motivation, and we can transmute its powerful energy into positive change in our lives.

But in order to bring about change we usually first need to believe that change is actually possible. However, this can sometimes become an irrelevance when we get swept up on a wave of change produced by discontent!

Strong dissatisfaction can become the catalyst for desirable change.

Permission to Succeed

By giving ourselves permission to fail we also give ourselves permission to succeed.

By granting ourselves the right to try, and to risk the possibility of failure, we are freed to take the necessary risks which ultimately produce our success.

However, from the perspective of higher meaning, there is no such thing as failure, only experience and growth.

Go for It

If you don't have a go,
you'll never know,
and if you don't begin,
then you can never win.

But even if you have been putting your life off,
remember, it's not how you start but how you
finish that really counts.

It is up to each and every one of us to make our
life really happen and if nothing is ever ventured
nothing can ever be gained.

This truly is your time.

So, take a deep breath, step into life and …
go for it.

Exploring New Lands

We can't explore life's wondrous oceans, or
venture to exciting new lands, until we discover
the courage to leave the shelter of the shore.

Opportunity

Opportunity is everywhere.

And if we believe opportunities abound, we will find them all around us. But if we believe no opportunities exist, we will not recognise them when they appear.

Sometimes we can miss our opportunities as they often come along heavily disguised as problems. In fact, an opportunity is often a solution to a presently prevailing problem, and the greater the size of the problem, the greater the opportunity. Examine carefully the problems of people and the world and there you will find rich opportunity. Find a need and fill it is the call.

All is possible. Inside each and every one of us is a wonderful creative genius which can generate new ideas, many of which can translate into exciting and rewarding realities. You don't have to be frustrated by waiting for opportunity to knock, you can step out boldly and create it.

Open your mind and be flexible; you are not limited.

---◆---

Success

We experience greater joy and fulfilment by
recognising that success is a journey.

If we believe success is just a destination, then we
miss all the joy along the way.

Success really is a journey.

So make the clear and unequivocal decision that
you are going to enjoy the trip.

Individual Creativity, not Competition

No-one can enjoy inner peace whilst seeing the world as a battlefield and everyone in it as competitors. Such an outlook will only keep us in a state of high alert – striving to stay ahead and fearful of falling behind.

In such a competitive world, others become viewed as our enemy instead of being loved as brothers and even someone else's failure can be the cause for celebration. But such competition only separates and divides.

Such fear-based competitive attitudes can be replaced by individual creativity, the uniquely personal expression of our distinctive talents and gifts. This way we avoid the anxiety which accompanies competition with others and free ourselves completely to admire the talents and abilities of all.

The challenge for us then becomes how best to express our uniqueness, so it provides us with meaning and purpose and best presents our gifts to the world.

Think Big

It is hard to catch big fish by staying in shallow waters. But push our boat into deeper waters and we place ourselves in better position to harvest the biggest catch.

It requires no major increase in effort and no greater output of energy to think big rather than small. But the difference in results can truly transform our lives.

Daring to trade our sparrow wings for powerful majestic eagle wings, we get to fly magically higher than we've ever flown before.

To elevate our lives we need firstly to elevate our thinking.

Excellence,
not Perfection

'The more we try to get close,
The more perfection recedes from our grasp.'

For many, many years, a man pursued the quality of perfection, believing he must acquire it to be whole. He chased it across high hills and into deep valleys, but always it was beyond his reach.

This made the man very unhappy as without the quality of perfection he felt distressed and incomplete.

One day, in emotional pain, he went to consult a famous healer. The healer told him that his problem was his vision – he needed to see both himself and his life in a different way. Then he gently rubbed the man's eyes and soon he could clearly see that he'd been pursuing an illusion, like an ever-receding shadow withdrawing before he arrived.

So, abandoning his search for perfection, he instead chose to settle for excellence and there discovered great satisfaction and a life of fulfilment and joy ...

Pursue excellence, not perfection.

Ideas for Wealth

Great ideas can produce great wealth. And we are invisibly but immutably connected to the source of all great ideas, like a sunbeam is joined to the sun.

However, ideas which generate great wealth do not demand that we reinvent the wheel but simply that we try to improve it by slightly changing its form in a way that serves our fellow man.

The Excellence Within

Contained within us all are seeds of greatness. For each and every one of us, there exists an area of excellence in which we can truly excel – the life work we are here to do.

Working in our field of excellence, we find a richly fulfilling expression which satisfies deep seated needs and adds purpose to our lives.

Our individual area of excellence will hold for us a fascination, a powerfully absorbing attraction, and above all it will bring us great joy as our work becomes a pleasure.

One of our major life tasks is to bring our gifts to the world, in a way that reflects our uniqueness and aligns with our highest calling.

Within us dwells the spark of divine purpose, which can ignite the human spirit into greatness.

Your Own Unique Journey

Following a life path which is not your own can produce conflict and unfulfilment. Living out a life of someone else's choosing can produce chronic dissatisfaction, resentment and strong regrets.

So, while it does make very good sense to take sound and wise counsel from others, always be prepared to travel your own unique and individual road.

Step out boldly in the direction of your dreams. Dare to paint your clouds green or colour your grass pink if such be your inspiration and calling. Take with you courage, determination and patience, making these your constant companions as each brings its own special magic.

Whatever your field of endeavour, live a life of loving service, discovering ever better ways of serving. Herein lies your greatest security.

Let your life be a true reflection of your highest and noblest nature, fitting snugly with your values like a hand in a tight-fitting glove.

Heart Work

By following your heart's guidance,
you inevitably will discover life's riches.

Doing the thing that you love is where your
treasure of fulfilment can be found.

A Wish

A wish is a desire without energy or power.

To manifest in our lives, a wish must be translated into strong and passionate desire, backed up and fully supported by a firmly committed decision.

Controlled and directed by the will, all then can be put in place through the use of an intelligent plan.

So, do not let your wishes die by floating aimlessly in the ether. Instead, harness your wish, give it clear direction and soon, through the power within you, it can become your new reality.

Clear Direction

Hour after hour in the hot sun, an ox toiled, pulling a mill wheel round and round. At the end of the day, it thought it had travelled a long way but in reality had been going round in circles, over and over the same old ground ...
In the absence of clear direction, how easy it can be to go round and round in circles, travelling the same old ground and eventually ending up where we really do not want to be.

We need to know, clearly and precisely, exactly where we want to go then create a plan to get there ... and determine to enjoy the trip.

Your Life Path

In the silence great things are fashioned, so take time to be still and listen.

Through the whispers of the heart and the impulse of desire, your Higher Power will tell you the life you are here to live.

Desire

'Inside each little acorn
is the desire to become a great oak.'

We all are infinitely creative and our deepest
heart's desires are the building blocks of all
we create.

Strong and passionate desire drives all our major
achievements, all our significant acquisitions. It is
the catalyst for our growth, a dynamic
motivational force causing us to be, have or do.

Our deepest heartfelt desires, those powerful
longings within, create an incompleteness, a
compelling unfilled need demanding to be met.

Rightful, virtuous desires seek only the good of all
and will never seek to cause harm to ourselves, to
others or the planet on which we live.

When an enduring virtuous desire has been
powerfully placed within us, the potential for its
attainment, at some level, already exists.
Empowered by this understanding, we can
confidently move ahead in the direction of
our dreams.

Aligned with higher purpose, that which you are
seeking is right now seeking you.

Determination

Determination and perseverance forge the steel of
self-belief and are a measure of your commitment
to the achievement of your goals.

The greater your resolution that you simply
won't be beaten, the greater the probability you
will succeed.

The Law of Attraction

'Like attracts like' is an immutable law of the Universe. Remember, each of us is just like a sunbeam eternally joined to the sun, invisibly, yet infinitely, connected to the unlimited source of all.

But to have what we want, we first must know what we want, ensuring that our desires truly reflect our higher nature. Then we can confidently lay our request upon the altar of our Higher Power, releasing and letting go, trusting it to handle the details. If it is in the interest of our highest good, that which we seek will manifest in a perfect way and in perfect time.

Simply hold the image of your desire clearly in your mind. Feel it strongly and impress it deeply. Live and breathe your heart's desire as though it was already yours. Then, step out courageously and boldly to do all that you must do.

Soon, like a living magnet, you'll discover you are on a collision course ... with the object of your desire.

Thoughts

Thoughts become things. Every building erected, every bridge designed, every book ever written, every business developed ... all began with thought.

Our thoughts of today create our reality of tomorrow – thoughts are causes, conditions are effects. For the most part, what we have and are today is very largely the product of our dominant thoughts from the past.

So, our power to think is also our power to create. When we control and master our thinking we gain mastery over our lives.

Thought is just like a seed which, planted in the mind and watered with strong conviction, eventually produces a harvest. Our lives in turn become just what our thoughts will make of it and, by choosing thoughts which are no longer limited, we create experiences which are no longer limited.

Keep your thoughts and your focus firmly on what you want for your life.

Wielding Power

'We sow the seeds each day of the tomorrows
we create.'

The Universe responds like one big cosmic
orchestra. And, just like a music conductor, we are
constantly wielding a baton directing the
symphony of our lives.

However, it's as though a screen is blocking our
vision and we can't see that the orchestra is there,
and neither do we understand how we influence
the end result. We casually scratch our nose and
violins begin to play. We find that when we raise
our arm the woodwind section starts up. We lean
to the right and the percussion comes alive.
Indeed, not knowing what's going on, or that we
actually direct it all, we may even recoil in horror
at the discordant cacophony of sound.

But by observing much more carefully, we can
eventually begin to see that the baton we wield so
influentially is the baton of our personal
consciousness, held in place by our thoughts and
underpinned by our beliefs …

Remember, our power to think is our power
to create.

The Imagination

The human imagination is an amazing instrument of power. Through our imagination, we fashion the future in advance: one of endless possibilities or one confined by limitation and constraint.

It is in the imagination, the creative workshop of the psyche, that we establish a blueprint of our destiny. Our powerful mental pictures, when combined with strong emotion, become etched upon the mind to form a point of reference as to what we can be, have or do.

And our powerful unconscious mind simply cannot tell the difference between what is actually real and what is vividly imagined. Unbridled 'negative' imagination can therefore wreak havoc in our lives.

To have the life we desire we must master the imagination. We need to keep it clearly focused on the things we want in life and away from what we do not want.

By keeping our imagination aligned with our desires, eventually we draw to us the image which we create.

The Law of Supply

By focusing on lack in our lives, we can imprint 'scarcity beliefs' and fill ourselves up with fear. However, when a lack appears to exist, this very often is a signal that we need to give something away. By learning to fearlessly give, we can demolish our walls of fear, opening up our access to supply.

If there is a lack of love in your life, give your love freely away. Seek nothing in return and, as you continue to generously give, you soon will unlock the floodgates and love will pour into your life.

Is it wealth you appear to lack? Then regularly give a little away to someone in greater need than yourself. As you become a loving giver, your faith and confidence will expand.

Through the act of fearlessly giving we conquer our fear of lack, establishing a consciousness of abundance and releasing our blocked supply.

Like attracts like and the giver attracts the gift.

An Abundant Universe

A master and his pupil observed, as a bird in the
garden fed on worms.
'The bird has come to teach you,' said the master.

As they watched, the bird performed its ritual:
tapping its foot on the ground, then tilting its
head from side to side. In a while, a worm would
emerge and the bird would eat its fill.

'What has this come to teach?' asked the pupil.

'First,' said the master, 'our supply is already there
though often hidden. But when the bird taps its
foot on the ground it attracts its supply to the
surface, as the worm thinks this is rain. Like the
bird, we also must take our "right action" to
attract and release our supply.'

'Lastly,' said the master, 'the reason the bird tilts
its head is that it listens for the movement of the
worm. So too we must be still and listen to know
where our gift can be found.'

Dream Great Dreams

Think great thoughts and dream great dreams.

A life without dreams is like a bird with broken wings – limited, confined and unable to fly.

Your great dream can fill you with passion to cross over your troubled waters and enter your promised land. Listen to your great dream, breathe life into it, let it deliver its precious gift to the world.

To make your great dream happen begin it boldly with courage and confidence. As you courageously stride towards your dream, it will also be travelling towards you and will meet you along the way.

Aim high. Shoot your visionary arrows at the stars. Even if they should miss, they'll still finish up in high and lofty places.

Taking Risks

Risks are mental training weights, ever expanding the muscles of courage, confidence and growth.

By seeking to avoid taking risks we may avoid rejection and pain, but the price that we must pay is very high. Without risks we cannot love. Without risks we cannot succeed. Without risks there is no growth or accomplishment of our dreams. Without risks we must forfeit real freedom. Chained to limitations, we become enslaved and imprisoned by the disempowering need to feel safe. Only through intelligent risks can we ever be truly free.

So take courage. Go to the edge of previous limitations and know that you can go beyond. Seek to fly a little higher than you've ever flown before. Soon you'll find yourself travelling to places you've never been to before.

Intelligent risks – and those full of growth – are the passport to becoming free.

A Secret of Success

One of the master secrets of success is determining the price you'll have to pay, then making a committed decision to be willing to pay that price.

Half measures rarely produce whole results. So, if something is worth doing, do it well. Do it with great passion, with conviction and enthusiasm, all wrapped in unstoppable persistence and determination to achieve your goal.

Seasons of Life

For everything there is a season and each fruit ripens in its own perfect time.

Recognising and accepting this truism, we can avoid the unnecessary struggle which comes when we resist the natural flow of life.

Inevitably, there may be times when we long for a change of season, however our anxious resistance and impatience can be just like trying to eat unripened fruit.

But we also must be alert to ensure that we do not sleep through our perfect time of harvest and opportunity.

Which season are you in right now? Is this your season for patient preparation? Or is right now your perfect time to reap, to gather in and enjoy the harvest you have already sown?

Consider which season you are in, then relax into your season.

'I Could' versus 'I Will'

There is a hugely significant difference between saying 'I could' and 'I will'.

'I could' is a statement of belief in our capacity to do something successfully. Unfortunately it falls far short of being a statement of intention to do it.

'I could' is our perceived potential and speaks of future possibilities, but it can subtly conceal inertia caused by fears and self-doubt. 'I could' can be a fantasy comforter, like a dream wish with no real power, and it can mask the unspoken words 'but sadly I never will'. 'I could', if not developed, can lead us deeply into the territory of frustrated and unrealised potential.

To harness our life possibilities, 'I could' must be developed and progressed to the next and vital stage of determinedly saying 'I will' – an unequivocal and clear cut decision with iron clad total commitment.

Money and Work

Money is inherently neither good nor bad, it is neutral. It is merely a means of exchange, and service is its source. The greater the service we render, the greater will be our return.

To increase the amount of money coming in, we can either increase the quantity or improve the quality of the service going out. Interestingly, by choosing to do more than we're paid for, often we soon will find we're being paid for more than we do.

Endeavour to perform all your work with a glad and joyous heart. However, if you are unable to give your service without resentment, perhaps you need to look closely at the work you presently do.

The more money that good people have, the more they are able to give. Placed in the right loving hands, money can do great things for humankind.

There certainly is nothing selfish about succeeding, then using your success to help create a better world.

Before Commencing

Before commencing any significant or highly
challenging task, pause for a moment of reflection.
Contemplate the effects of the totally completed
task ... and then begin.

This way you'll find it easier to accomplish. And as
your work will then carry greater meaning, it
inevitably will produce higher levels of satisfaction.

Expectations

Try always to keep your expectations positive. Your
expectations for yourself should be sufficiently
high to challenge you, but also realistic and
achievable so you don't become discouraged or
overwhelmed. Unrealistic expectations can lead to
major letdowns and can be a major source of
distress, often diminishing the likelihood
of success.

Set your self-expectations at incremental levels
which have a sound possibility of achievement
given appropriate application and effort combined
with a positive, enthusiastic approach.

Killing Time

One extremely cold night in the desert, a travelling Arab merchant was begged by his camel to let it warm just its nose in his tent. Reluctantly the merchant agreed.

But very soon the camel had eased its head into the tent, then its front legs, next the humps. Eventually it took over the tent and drove the merchant out into the cold.

The name of this camel was Procrastination.

Procrastination is not just the thief of time, it also is the robber of achievement. Just like the camel, it can take us over a little at a time, driving our will out into the cold.

Each time we postpone our actions we rob ourselves of power. Simultaneously we are weakening our will.

So, whatever you must do, begin it boldly, begin it now. Make time your friend, not your enemy. Treat it with great respect.

Remember, if we choose to kill time, we risk murdering our success.

The Energy of Success

It takes as much mental energy to fail,
as it actually does to succeed.

But the principal difference in results
lies in where that energy is placed.

Taking Life's
Short Cuts

Perched upon a tree in a forest, a bird was singing cheerful songs when along came a man with a box of succulent worms.

'I'll give you a worm for just one of your feathers,' the man shouted to the bird.

The bird thought for a while. Then it decided that this really seemed much easier than flying around the forest in search of its daily food. So several times every day the bird would exchange a feather for a juicy worm.

Then, some weeks later, the bird suddenly and painfully discovered that it could no longer fly. To make matters even worse, it now felt so unattractive that it simply no longer felt able to sing its cheerful songs...

Often the promised 'short cut' can prove to be too expensive. If something is worth having or doing we need to be prepared to pay the full and rightful price.

Beware the short-term gain which could result in long-term pain.

Delaying Gratification

As any significant achievement will require significant effort, it is important to develop the ability to put off the experience of pleasure, to delay our gratification.

In the interests of our long-term gain we must endure some short-term pain such as discipline, application and effort. Even the greatest of inspirations still calls for some perspiration.

Developing skill, expertise or knowledge, or achieving any major accomplishment, will take time. We therefore need to learn to be patient. And by learning to stay focused on the process we can avoid overwhelming ourselves, which unfortunately can sometimes happen when we become fixated on the end result and the size of the overall task.

But with practice we can come to experience the wonderful sacredness of now and begin to happily achieve. Step by gentle step, we can move in the direction of our dream, fulfilling our appointment with destiny.

Take pleasure in delaying gratification in the interests of your highest good.

Valuing the Prize

When something comes to us without any effort,
it can easily slip through our hands.

But when we have to strive hard to acquire it,
we more greatly value the prize.

Failure Seeds

The story is told of an ancient destructive spirit whose major duty it was to destroy achievement and fulfilment in human lives. The name of this destructive spirit was the Life Robber.

One day, the Life Robber put on display his instruments of human struggle. There, laid out for viewing, were many of his destructive tools: envy, hatred, greed, malice, selfishness, and many, many more.

But, set aside from all the others, was one particularly powerful instrument he used extensively in human defeat. The name of this destructive tool was discouragement.

Discouragement is particularly powerful because on first viewing it seems so inoffensive, yet once it has become established it lets in all the rest.

Be aware and say 'no' to discouragement, the destroyer of achievement and fulfilment. Take courage and know deep inside that you can succeed.

Honest Toil

Better to do a humble, but honest, day's toil than to play the part of a rich man ... and go hungry.

Great wealth can never totally protect the rich but harsh abject poverty can readily destroy the poor. Be a generous and loving giver to those less fortunate than yourself.

Indecision

A hungry but indecisive mule stood between two bales of hay, simply unable to decide from which of the bales it would eat. On either side of the mule lay an abundant supply of food, but it kept constantly wavering, unable to make up its mind. Submerged in total confusion, it eventually weakened and died ...

A season of reflective thinking can be helpful to sort out our concerns and enable us to arrive at a more decisive state of mind. But an excessive reflective season can become disempowerment and confusion through protracted hesitation and doubt and a failure to make up our mind.

A split and divided mind can begin to lose its power and weaken, just like a fractured limb. Often, a clear and very definite decision will renew and restore our lost power.

Discover the power of decision.

Share your Success

Be sure to give yourself adequate time to relax and enjoy your success.

And seek to share that same success with those who have helped along the way. There is nothing quite so empty or lonely as arriving at the pinnacle of achievement and finding yourself there on your own.

So, let loving people fill your world. Not only will they be able to share your success, but the more people there are in your life, the more hands there will be to catch you, if ever you should find that you fall.

Christen Everything Success

We all are students in this game of life, placed upon the planet to learn and grow.

Viewed from this perspective, as long as we learn from every situation, then there is no such thing as failure, only experience and continuous growth.

And success is certainly not limited to those who come in first – we can successfully come in tenth when we finished twelfth last time. When the primary goal has been established *to participate, to evolve and to grow*, then as long as we're moving forward we are succeeding every time.

Providing we learn from each situation, we can christen everything success.

Our Mission

Our mission is to bring beauty, goodness and love
to the world in our own unique and special way.

And to reach out to heal the love famine
of humanity's starving heart.

The Gifts You Bring to the World

You may bring to the world the gift of your compassion, to tenderly enfold the pain of humankind.

Or you might share with the world the gift of your generous nature. How the Universe really loves a kind and generous giver!

Maybe your gift to the world is the vision of the reformer, seeking to put right the injustice that you find.

Perhaps you offer to the world the gift of a patient listener, to help heal the wounds and fractures of broken human lives.

A special offering to the world is being a beloved mother or father, guiding and nurturing your children to give them strength for future days.

But whatever other gifts you offer, the most priceless gift of all is to be your own truly unique person, offering the world the gift of your authentic loving self.

The Love Centre Within

Deep within us is a centre of pure love. We all know or at least sense that it is there, but often we deny its existence.

However, what we do not recognise is that this love centre within us is dynamic. It is constantly at work on our behalf, cajoling, fashioning, manoeuvring, all the while conspiring to serve us, to heal our lives and make us whole.

At times we may hear its whispers, calling us to live with love, but sadly we may reject the call. And when we resist these promptings to love, we experience the uncomfortable feelings of not being in our rightful place.

Whatever is going on in our lives, or however dark our past has been, this love within will never leave us. It always will be there, loving and supporting us, because this love is *us*, it is our Higher Self.

We never lose the love option for our lives – the door to love is always open wide.

The Oneness of All

A wise master took his pupil to the woods to teach him of the oneness of all.

Breaking a seed from a tree, the master said, 'If I plant this seed and another tree grows, is not the second tree part of the first? If I then take a seed from the second tree and with it grow yet another, is the third tree not also part of both the first and second trees?'

He continued, 'And should I grow a whole forest of trees, has not the first tree then become all? And does it not exist within all? Though each tree might believe itself separate, are they all not eternally joined? And should the first tree no longer exist, does it not forever live in all the other trees?'

All that has gone before lives on in each new creation. Our separateness is an illusion. There is no separation in divine mind ... we all are eternally joined.

Making Sense of the Divine

As we look around our planet, at times we may become confused as we earnestly and sincerely struggle to make sense of a world with God. But how impossible it can become to extract real meaning and purpose from a life that does not contain God.

By recognising the liberating simplicity contained within 'God is love' we can look at the love all around us and see our Higher Power everywhere. Following on from this simple definition, all that is not love is also not of God.

When we think and act with love, we are perfectly in tune with the infinite, co-creating with our Higher Power.

Returning to Source

One of the deepest pains we can endure is the pain of chronic emptiness. Whilst we all desire to experience fulfilment, we may instead feel empty inside.

And there is within us all an instinctive urge to wholeness, to the unity of completion. We long to know a deeper connectedness, a higher sense of belonging.

The hollow pain or emptiness we may feel can be the pain of separation from our source, the pain of separation from love. In fact, the whole of our life is a journey which eventually leads us back to love, just like a salmon returning to its source.

Wholeness and completion are found when we join in a mystical union and our lives become one with love. Indeed, love itself is our essential nature and we finally step out of pain by becoming one with the love that we are.

The call is to return to love, to make the expression of unconditional love the primary focus of our lives.

Create your own Epitaph

To depart the planet in peace,
determine the epitaph you desire.

Then set out to live a life which creates it.

Your Life Makes
a Difference

At this precise moment in time, without your
loving presence our planet would not be complete.
You are here upon the Earth because you are
meant to be here and your life does make
a difference.

The consciousness of humankind is like one huge
spreading tree covered with countless green leaves.
But should just one leaf turn red, it changes the
form of the tree.

So too with the consciousness of humanity. The
thoughts, the deeds and attitudes of each and
every person impacts upon the whole. Every kindly
act, every loving thought, each compassionate
word is just like a leaf turning red on the
consciousness of humankind.

We are here to create the virtuous, the beautiful
and the good, so use your gifts well to make this a
better world.

Your life does make a difference and this world is
made richer by your loving presence.

Your Earth Journey

As you travel your Earth journey ...
Be all that you can be,
do the best that you can do.

Learn what you're here to learn,
teach what you're here to teach.

Give all that you can give,
help all whom you can help.

Love, as best you can, without conditions.

Let your joy and laughter fill the air
as you learn to live from the heart
and to sing your own special song.

Forgive all, do not envy, do not blame.

Take time to smell the roses,
appreciate the smaller things in life.

And in your own unique way,
leave your footprint on the planet.

The End

The end is but a new beginning.

Personal Growth Training

Bill Longridge presents a range of Personal Growth Training programmes for groups and organisations.

These include:

Out of Pain into Power

Discover your Magnificent Self

The Gift of Self-Esteem

Developing Super Self-Confidence

Overcoming the Fear of Making Presentations

For information on these and other training programmes, please write to the author via the publisher.

Bill Longridge is home based in both Ireland and Australia; however, courses can be provided in any English-speaking country.